I Once Was Fat but Now I'm Found:

Part 1 – First Steps to Food Freedom

by Laura Fulford

I Once Was Fat but Now I'm Found: Part 1 – First Steps to Food Freedom

Written by Laura Fulford

Copyright Laura Fulford 2019.

All rights reserved.

Published 2019.

ISBN: 9781797548678

Scripture quotations are from The ESV® Bible (The Holy Bible, English Standard Version®), copyright © 2001 by Crossway, a publishing ministry of Good News Publishers. Used by permission. All rights reserved.

"For freedom Christ has set us free; stand firm therefore, and do not submit again to a yoke of slavery."
- Galatians 5:1

"So, whether you eat or drink, or whatever you do, do all to the glory of God."
- I Corinthians 10:31

Contents

Introduction	7
Chapter One: The Search for the Skinny Grail	17
Chapter Two: Needles and Impossible Passageways	25
Chapter Three: What's in Your Closet?	31
Chapter Four: Who's Your Daddy?	59
Chapter Five: Help!	93
Final Word	119
Notes	121
About the Author	123

Introduction

In Autumn of 1969, a group of boys and girls frolicked on a grassy front yard in a suburban North Florida neighborhood. Football season had begun. The yard had shifted from imaginary diamond to gridiron accordingly.

We were getting down to business; picking teams and assigning players to offensive or defensive roles. I anticipated being one of the first girls picked, having several advantages: my big brothers were the team organizers, it was my parents' front yard, and I was willing to play the thankless position of center.

On this otherwise typical day, as I was bouncing around in carefree pre-adolescent energy, I noticed one boy's gaze had fixed on me. He appeared to be gripped by a vision he couldn't quite grasp. Time slowed down as his face contorted and these words emerged from his disgusted little lips: "You're fat!"

That is my earliest and most palpable memory of the heart-sting of shame. This pint-sized human conveyed verbally and non-verbally that he found my appearance entirely displeasing. His noticeable visceral reflex left a deeper impression than his words. *I must be quite hideous*, I concluded.

Like Eve, who on that fateful day in the garden suddenly saw her own nakedness, my eyes were also opened. I saw myself, and like Eve, I felt the intense desire to hide and cover myself. My new concerns became body image and dieting.

As luck would have it, my mother was a yo-yo dieter. I took subtle cues from her that being overweight is, indeed, a problem. Menu adjustments would be needed. My thin older brother got the cupcakes; I got the celery sticks.

Occasionally, my father expressed his concern about my size more overtly. The older I got, the harder it became for him to refrain from helping me see that being fat would be a handicap for me in life. Sadly, it did affect our relationship, even though his intentions were for my good.

That childhood incident left me wary of future occurrences. Upon seeing me, people might recoil reflexively. And I, noticing, would feel ashamed and want to hide. Hiding my excess weight had serious limitations. I was too young for heels and too round for vertical stripes to work their slimming magic. There was no quick fix short of reincarnation (which would have been nice, but I knew not to bank on it.) What's a girl to do? I resigned myself to living on alert.

My little football friend was the first of many more who couldn't refrain from commenting on my appearance. In third grade, during a lesson about face shapes, one teacher's assistant sauntered past four or five of my kid-colleagues, right to where I was sitting. She looked straight at me and said, "YOUR face is ROUND." As she said it, she drew a circle with her finger, outlining my face, like I might not understand had she not added that helpful non-verbal cue. *Gee, thanks, but I'm just fat, not stupid.* I smiled at her, acknowledging her observation, but hid my hurt feelings.

As a teenager, my weight limited—or rather, eliminated—social opportunities, including dating, and milestone events, such as the prom. In my 20's, a male co-worker said to me, "You aren't fat; you just have an odd shape." *Really? I feel so much better now.*

One of the most difficult encounters to forget was one with my father. My 20s were challenging. I doubted myself and all the decisions I had made. I had trouble finding a job. One day, as I stood in the kitchen eating, my father approached me and said, "Men don't hire fat women, and women don't hire fat women." Then, he walked away. I doubt he liked saying it any more than I liked hearing it.

He and I both attributed all my problems to my weight. We both saw it as the one thing that stood in the way of everything worth having in life. We both gave my weight more power than it ever deserved.

Shame over my size made me hypersensitive to people's reactions. I swore I could see it—that moment when my appearance hit their visual cortex and registered "Whoa! She's fat!" I was convinced everyone was judging me, whether they were or not. I longed for the day when my size and shape wouldn't be the first, or perhaps only, thing someone would notice about me. Why did I feel as though I owed the world an apology for showing up "like this?"

Conspiracy to Commit Denial

Amidst the pain of being overweight, you'd think I would "get it" that my eating was a contributing factor. It wasn't that I didn't know. I simply couldn't face it. Perhaps it's the addict's dilemma. The "drug" that gives momentary pleasure, relief from pain and escape from reality, only digs you in deeper and causes you more pain in the long run. Like an addict, I avoided facing the obvious and convinced myself I could overpower it.

I tried to hide my habit like a good magician hides an airplane. How do you hide a big problem? Produce a slightly larger diversion. My "go-to" diversions were:

- Bad genes...
- Slow metabolism...

The diversions allowed me (in my mind) to deflect judgment about my size and attention away from what I ate. Heaven forbid anyone should think I ate too much. That was a level of exposure I couldn't bear thinking about. I even avoided eating in front of people.

The Land of Misfit Diets

For decades, I dieted, and broke diets, lost and gained, over and over through grade school, high school, college, and beyond. I tried every diet there was, or some form of it. I tried several other options as well.

In college, I majored in Exercise Science, thinking that if I had a career in health and fitness, I would surely conquer my weight problem. I did learn how I could theoretically conquer a weight problem. I could tell you how to do it in unpronounceable detail. And even though I was "fit" from exercising fiercely for four hours a day, I still carried varying degrees of extra weight.

Before "exercise bulimia" had a label, I was a card carrier. I was convinced I could "work off" more than I ate. I dedicated hours each day to some form of exercise. I taught step aerobics, lifted weights, played tennis, swam laps, and took up biking. The results? No weight lost. Next, I resorted to running. Runners are thin, I observed. Running long distances was going to be my missing link. I ran more and more, participating in various races, including two marathons. I learned a valuable lesson. Thin runners are, indeed, thin. Other runners, like me, were not. When my extra weight held on stubbornly through two years of training for and running two marathons, it was time to get serious: liposuction.

Liposuction was...interesting. The serious physical pain and enormous expense made for a relatively effective appetite suppressant. The vice-like post-surgical corset I had to wear around my midsection made it hard to breathe, much less to eat. Yes, I lost some weight, but this, too, was temporary.

As a side note, one *can* gain weight after liposuction. Of course, I gained it in areas that weren't suctioned, such as my arms, neck, and those lateral flaps just above my bra line that I referred to as my bat wings.

By the time I hit 40 years-old, it had dawned on me that my weight might not be the problem, but rather, a symptom.

The Prodigal Dieter

For all those years, I indulged my self-deception as often as I indulged my cravings. I purposely avoided God the way a dog avoids his master after gnawing her favorite shoes.

My relationship with God was an amalgamation of things I'd learned in Christian elementary school and years of church with a smattering of meaning well and trying hard, for the most part. My "theology" rested on the foundation of a prayer I had repeated when I was 9 years old. I had never really had a reason to test my theology or my faith for its soundness.

Turning to God made me apprehensive, like going to the dentist to examine an achy tooth. Would this be painful? Considering all the years of failure and frustration, I asked myself, *how much worse could it get?* I eased in, poking around to see how other Christians were dealing with this issue.

To my surprise, there were many "Bible-based" programs to explore, more than I had imagined. I sat through a few Bible studies about weight loss and even facilitated a few. Many Christian women shared my struggle. I noticed a familiar pattern among us. We all enjoyed the studies. We loved the Bible reading, we prayed, we enjoyed meeting together, but none of us were losing weight.

Here again was the same pattern as in any other diet program. Just like the rest of the world, we Christians were gaining and losing the same half pound repeatedly, or gaining even more weight. I might have accumulated five more pounds in the process.

Why wouldn't daily doses of Bible reading and prayer do the trick? What are a few pounds to the God who created the world and parted the Red Sea? We engaged in spiritual disciplines on top of dieting and exercising. So, why wasn't God rewarding us with steady weight loss? No, we weren't doing the diet and exercise perfectly. That would be too legalistic. We didn't want rules; we wanted grace, freedom, and shrinking fat cells, not necessarily in that order. When I peeked through the Christian veneer, this was no different than any other program. We were Christians wanting the same things as anybody else and experiencing the same defeats as anybody else.

A few of us broke ranks, got real, and called the emperor naked. We admitted we were acting like God was the Wizard of Oz. But instead of courage, heart, and brains, we wanted tiny waists, skinny thighs, and firm buttocks. We were hoping that just the right verse, if memorized and repeated enough times, would work like a nicotine patch, or in my case, a chocolate chip cookie patch.

Diagnosis: Mortal

I never did find a "patch" in the Bible, but I did find a diagnosis. I don't remember a passage ever landing harder on my heart. In Romans 7, the Apostle Paul revealed the nature of my illness. He wrote, *"For I do not understand my own actions. For I do not do what I want, but I do the very thing I hate... So I find it to be a law that when I want to do right, evil lies close at hand. For I delight in the law of God, in my inner being, but I see in my members another law waging war against the law of my mind and making me captive to the law of sin that dwells in my members. Wretched man that I am! Who will deliver me from this body of death?"* (selected verses from Romans 7:15-24).

The diagnosis? I was unable to stop myself from overeating. I wanted to, but I couldn't. I needed help. I need someone to deliver me. If Paul was experiencing this conundrum, I knew I was dealing with something way beyond my capability. I didn't have a weight problem, or a food problem. I had a spiritual problem. It was my first tangible introduction to my flesh nature.

In Romans 7 and 8, Paul revealed the cure and an entirely new set of questions. *"Thanks be to God through Jesus Christ our Lord! So then, I myself serve the law of God with my mind, but with my flesh I serve the law of sin. There is therefore now no condemnation for those who are in Christ Jesus. For the law of the Spirit of life has set you free in Christ Jesus from the law of sin and death"* (Romans 7:25-8:3). I needed the Spirit to set me free. Why wasn't I free already? I had to ask, Lord —what does *that* mean? How does *that* work?

The answer came when I realized that I wasn't serving Him. I was asking Him to serve me, to help me lose weight, to help me look the way I wanted. The Spirit of Jesus couldn't set me free if I wasn't willing to give Him the freedom He needed to work in my life the way He wanted to instead of the way I wished He would.

Spanning nearly four decades, I left a vapor trail of failed weight loss experiments. I often regret spending so much time and emotion chasing my tail. Only Christ can redeem the time and opportunities I lost. God has a very kind and merciful way of redeeming our lives and the foibles that comprise them. My prayer is that His redemption flows through my story and the lessons I gathered along this path that many women have walked and maybe are still walking, wondering where the exit is.

I Once Was Fat

There are endless things to learn about losing weight. If you're like me, you'll be tempted to think that finding THE one thing and then doing THAT is the answer.

For some people, maybe all they need is a little more information. For others, no matter what they do, or how valiantly they fight, the war never ends. I was the latter kind.

This book is for people like me: Christians who battle against a stronghold. If diets and exercise resolve the issue for you, maybe your challenge is just physical. But if you've tried everything only to fall defeated again and again, then, perhaps, it's time to look deeper; what's going on mentally, emotionally, spiritually?

This book is part 1 in a series aimed at helping Christians stop fighting the wrong battle. Yes, food is involved, but it's not just about the food. Weight is involved, but weight is only a symptom, not the problem. It's about more than losing weight; it's about freedom. We can't be free in Christ when we are enslaved in a stronghold. Let's look at how to start on the path to freedom, leaving behind the stronghold of weight and food and moving toward real freedom in Christ as our Lord.

I'm praying you will find:

- Hope and encouragement from a sister who has been enslaved *and* delivered,

- Real transformation from the only One who genuinely transforms the human heart.

- His power to overcome.

May you have nothing short of His supernatural sanctifying work in your life. His work is the only work that can truthfully be called "transformational."

Envision your life in Christ as you leave behind your weight struggle. God wants to free us to walk in the works He ordained in advance for our lives. He has plans for you.

> *"For we are His workmanship, created in Christ Jesus for good works, which God prepared beforehand that we should walk in them."*
> *- Ephesians 2:10*

Chapter One:
The Search for the Skinny Grail

As a diet enlightened 6-year-old, I entered the world of weight obsession. Out with Coca Cola, in with Tab. Out with Swiss Rolls, in with Melba Toast and its gnarly cousin, Wasa bread.

Starting so young, I fancy myself a time-tested in-the-trenches researcher. I've devoured hundreds of diet books, often while gnawing on a piece of pizza. My findings? The elusive secret I hoped for, the "Holy Grail of weight loss," was nowhere to be found. There had to be *something* that would make losing weight easy. This magic potion would kill my appetite for sweets, or it would give me the will to do what was required —forever. I was on a quest, nose to the ground like a bloodhound.

I cut my teeth on Stillman, Atkins, Pritikin, The Grapefruit Diet, The (unofficial) Mayo Clinic Diet, and Weight Watchers, to name a few. The list grew year by year. My sister would often join me to follow some ridiculous plans. One of them involved eating 48 eggs over a period of two weeks and enough spinach to burst Popeye's biceps.

Every new diet played out in the same pattern: I would lose a few pounds and then start bending the rules. While on Weight Watchers, I ate my allotted 22 points (give or take) in *Doritos* and Rocky Road ice cream. On Atkins, after I got sick of chicken, steak, and bacon, I shifted to cream cheese and chocolate covered macadamia nuts. I ended up in diet Hades, that nightmarish place where one tells herself (and others) she is dieting, but mysteriously still gaining weight.

I was determined to unearth an explanation (that exonerated me) for my weight loss conundrum. Perhaps a rare birth defect or an interruption in the time-space continuum was to blame. As a young woman with an Exercise Science degree and the entire "Healthy Living" section of *Barnes and Noble* on my bookshelves, I had convinced myself it *couldn't* be my fault.

Losing weight is indeed trickier than it appears. It's like a shell game. It presents itself as a physical problem (how much we weigh) and points to an "obvious" solution (diet and exercise). But if that were true, wouldn't there be *scientific* evidence that diet and exercise lead to success? Do a little digging, and you'll discover losing weight and keeping it off is rare. Less than five percent of people who lose weight keep the weight off long term.[1] Digesting that statistic, I witnessed it was true of me and true of most people I knew who also struggled with their weight. My chronic weight loss failure was common and predictable. Even so, I wasn't comforted.

In my 35+ years of dieting experience, I estimate that my net gain/loss is close to 1,000 pounds. Many have told me they share this experience: decades of dieting and herculean efforts with exercise, losing weight, gaining it back, rinse, repeat. I had proven one thing to myself: there is more to it than diet and exercise. But my trail had grown cold, as had my willingness to punish myself with diets any more. Maybe the problem was in my head. I expanded the circle of my search.

The Salad Fork in the Road

Behavioral psychology was a new trail for me to bark down, sniffing for the missing link in my weight journey. Could there be a solution that had nothing to do with dry salad or distance running? Apparently, my prior approach was lacking. I'd failed to consider the part of my body above my mouth. I was all horse, no cart. All grit, no wit. I shifted to the psychology section of the book store. Perhaps all along what I needed was to be off the treadmill and on the counselor's couch.

Is it surprising that humans struggle with change, especially achieving long-term change? The anecdotal evidence is everywhere. Permanent weight loss is a type of long-term change. Like the other types, such as quitting smoking, drinking, gambling, pornography, etc., we rarely succeed. Clinical studies reveal that most of us are unlikely to pull ourselves out of these patterns, even when we desperately want to.

Change isn't simple. It's more like a Rubik's Cube, less like a light switch. Many scientists have devoted their lives to unveiling why so few people successfully change bad habits. For the ones that do change, how did they escape self-destructive behavior patterns? They clearly had a secret and were keeping it from the rest of us. I was dying to find out. My voyage of discovery was getting interesting. Would it lead me to the secret to permanent weight loss?

One human change theory garnered my attention like a coupon for free cake mix: the Transtheoretical Model of Change, or TTM for short. For a girl in search of a tasty excuse for my food/weight predicament, it had me at *Transtheoretical*. Was this the needle in the haystack? I grabbed a magnifying glass and dove in looking for the "off switch" to my inner brownie eater.

The study observed 1,000 people who had stopped smoking, drinking, and overeating for years. They were like the spotted owls of weight loss—rare, and precious. How did they do it? What would their patterns reveal? Could we follow in their skinny little footsteps?

Sure enough, there were patterns. The study resulted in a detailed explanation of the six very "sciencey" sounding phases of change. The details are in the book, *Changing For Good*.[1] Apparently, these 1,000 people had spiraled their way through these phases of change, three steps forward, two steps back until they broke their habits for good, and for years and years to follow.

Was there a breadcrumb here for me? Could this lead me to success? Could it, at least, explain my failure? I hadn't considered the psychological complexity of change, or considered my mind was the subversive party. Yet there I was on the wrong part of the chart.

The phases are summarized in the chart below.

Phase	Mindset
1. Pre-contemplation	"I can't do it," or "I won't do it."
2. Contemplation	"I might do it."
3. Preparation	"I will do it."
4. Action	"I am doing it."
5. Maintenance	"I am still doing it."
6. Termination	"Look, Mom, no hands!"

I was wedged between phase 1 and phase 2. Most of the time, my mind was saying "no" or "let me get back to you on that." My mind was unwilling to commit to my hopes and plans. It was like trying to get socks on a disgruntled toddler.

This was, indeed, a new insight. I remained uninspired to throw out my back up stash of brownie mix, but, at least, I had a new name for my "condition." I was a "chronic contemplator," always considering action but not following through. It was a refreshing addition to my "slow metabolism" excuse.

This psychological model described (in more detail than I needed) what I knew by experience:

- Change is genuinely hard.
- Most people don't make it.
- Humans are complicated; it's messy under the hood.

Why I hadn't spiraled my way to maintenance remained a mystery. I was one of the masses that didn't, not one of the few that did.

On the bright side, these new insights pointed me to new questions. Why wasn't my deep desire to be thin enough to carry me to my ideal weight?

Reflections

Have you ever wrestled with similar questions? Have you wondered why your desire to lose weight feels so strong but can't seem to carry you long-term?

This was one of the questions that prompted me to stop avoiding the Lord and turn, albeit slightly, toward Him. I presented myself to Him as I was: defeated. Broken. Frustrated. He had been waiting wisely, graciously, patiently, lovingly. He was about to open my eyes.

Questions

Feel free write your answers in your book. You can also print these questions from StopDietingforLife.com.

1. What experiences of yours come to your mind as you read this chapter?

2. Recall some of the diets and weight loss plans you have tried. Does knowing the complicated nature of change influence your perspective? If so, how?

3. Have you ever felt reluctant to take steps you ought to take? Describe your hesitation. (It can be hard to pinpoint, but do your best.)

4. Take a few minutes now and pray. Record your prayer.

Chapter Two:
Needles and Impossible Passageways

I don't recall the first time I tasted something sweet. I also can't recall ever *not* having the urge to eat something sweet.

My childhood best friend was also named Laura. I was 3 years old, and she was 2 when her family moved in across the street. We became inseparable. Laura was always thin. On the weight bell curve, we resided on opposite ends of the bubble. The only thing that separated us was approximately 6 standard deviations.

At my house, my mom kept the cookies on the top shelf, (literally) out of my sight and reach. Laura's mom kept awesome snacks right where we could see them. Sweet treats were restricted at my house, but the ease of obtaining a fix at Laura's house was always on my radar screen. She couldn't have cared less about snacks. An MRI of my brain would reveal a box of Blueberry Pop-Tarts.

As Laura and I grew older, she remained thin. I continued to be quite overweight and quite distressed by it. My deepest desires—to eat without restraint and to be thin—were in a perpetual smackdown. I resigned myself to the perpetual inner conflict, as one might adjust to chronic tinnitus.

My food or my figure —one of those was going to win. The food had always won, undefeated. My figure made an occasional run at victory, only to be crushed at the 1-yard line. I wanted them both to win —like those people who eat like fullbacks but look like ballerinas. I wasn't interested in alternative outcomes.

What Must I Do?

In Matthew 19:23-24, Jesus said to His disciples, *"Truly, I say to you, only with difficulty will a rich person enter the kingdom of heaven. Again I tell you, it is easier for a camel to go through the eye of a needle than for a rich person to enter the kingdom of God."*

Even the disciples sometimes looked at each other and whispered, "What does He mean?" As I read these words, I knew Jesus was speaking to me.

What prompted Jesus to say this, that rich people were more likely headed for an unpleasant eternal surprise? His words came on the heels of a conversation with a privileged young man—think Prince Harry but Jewish. The young man asked Jesus about eternal life, and perhaps some validation of his good life. Was he on the right track? He asked Jesus, *"Teacher, what good deed must I do to have eternal life?"* (Matthew 19:16). The young man explained to Jesus that he had faithfully kept the commandments since he was young. Was there anything more he should do to assure himself a place in Heaven?

Knowing the young man's heart, Jesus told him to give his wealth to the poor and to come follow Him. *What?* Jesus had just asked him to do what was inconceivable for him. Impossible.

The young man was crestfallen. How could he leave his life, his wealth, and his position to follow Jesus? This was not a simple choice. It was the ultimate choice: which had greater value to him, now or eternity? Himself or God?

Jesus had not so subtly revealed a commandment of God the young man had not been able to keep: *"You shall have no other gods before me"* (Exodus 20:3).

The young man wasn't looking for God or Jesus the Messiah. He was looking for eternal life on his own terms. He wanted eternal life to "work" the way he had been banking on all his life. He wanted Heaven. Would it have mattered to him whether Jesus was there or not? If it didn't matter when Jesus stood right there, why would it matter in eternity? *Would it matter to me?*

Ironically, Eternal Life stood right smack in front of this man and spoke to him, but the young man couldn't see Him. He could only see what he wanted. Validation was all he wanted from Jesus. He didn't want the Truth. He certainly didn't want what he got.

As I processed the scene of the young man walking away sad, I wondered, *What just happened?* Was Jesus asking him to give up all he owned? Was Jesus saying he had to choose between eternal life and a life of wealth? What was Jesus *really* asking?

The disciples were no less puzzled and alarmed. In Matthew 18:25, they asked Jesus, *"Then who can be saved?"* Jesus answered in verse 26 and offered hope to what seemed like an impossible situation. *"What is impossible with man is possible with God."*

Jesus' encounter with this young man landed hard on my heart. I was in a similar place —unprepared and unwilling to offer the kind of surrender Jesus was proposing. No, I wasn't a wealthy princess. But I knew in my heart that if I was standing in that man's sandals, I would meet the same impasse. *I'll do anything, Lord, except...*

The story wasn't new to me. Jesus had also delivered the same message in other situations. Why was it only now rattling my cage? Was it the gravity of the choice?

"Then Jesus said to his disciples, 'Whoever wants to be my disciple must deny themselves and take up their cross and follow me. [25] For whoever wants to save their life will lose it, but whoever loses their life for me will find it. [26] What good will it be for someone to gain the whole world, yet forfeit their soul? Or what can anyone give in exchange for their soul?'" Matthew 16:24-26

If I couldn't honestly say yes to His call to follow Him, what did that say about my faith? My relationship with Him? Was I His disciple? What did this even mean about my salvation?

At the very least, I needed to understand it better, and why I felt the tightness in my heart of a spiritual impasse. What was it that I wouldn't lay down to follow Him? For the young ruler, it was deeper than wealth. For me, it went deeper than the food and my longing to be thin.

In my "Rich Young Ruler" moment with Jesus, I was gripped. Uncomfortable. Squirming. I felt the young man's dilemma. What Jesus was asking of him was impossible for him. Was He also asking the impossible of me? Would I walk away sad, as the young ruler did? Had I done that already, over and over?

Camel Meets Needle

My spiritual impasse was unsettling. After trying, I learned I couldn't simply snap out of it. I couldn't "wish away" my resistance to surrender my life to Jesus. What choice was I facing? It wasn't as clear then as it is now. But I knew I didn't want to follow Jesus more than I wanted my life the way I wanted it. I had invested all my hopes and desires in what I thought my life would be like if I was thin. That had become what I lived to pursue. In fact, I wanted Jesus to help me achieve that end.

What response was Jesus asking me for? A much bigger change of heart, one I couldn't make on my own, and honestly, didn't even want to make. What does a girl do when something is needed, required, but way beyond her ability?

This must be that camel/needle conundrum Jesus was referencing. I didn't have a diet book or a psychological manual to fall back on for this one. I needed Jesus to make the impossible possible in my heart in a way that I had no control over, no ability, and not a lot of desire to make happen.

The Lord knew what to do. He was leading me here. He brought me through a process that I call the **Spiritual Model of Change** for two reasons. First, it picked me up where the psychological model of change left me looking up and thinking, *Lord, —no human can explain the complexity You built into us. There is so much more to this than psychology*. Second, it's a process with many steps, not an on-off switch. These steps guided me into His saving and sanctifying work in my heart.

The model describes the way God helped me through my spiritual impasse. He met me where I was and untangled me from this enslaving battle so that I could follow Him with sincerity of heart.

The Spiritual Model of Change

The Spiritual Model of Change unfolds in three phases, with a few steps in each phase. Here is an outline to help you follow along as we walk through each part in the next chapters:

1. *Looking Inward (Chapter Three)*
    a. *Explore*
    b. *Be Honest*
    c. *Count the Cost*
    d. *Realize*
2. *Looking to God (Chapter Four)*
    a. *Believe*
    b. *Trust*
    c. *Honor*
    d. *Offer*
3. *Looking to Community (Chapter 5)*

Chapter Three:
What's in Your Closet?

Within each phase of the Spiritual Model of Change are several small steps. Each will help you to prepare your heart to follow Jesus away from what enslaves you. This chapter will cover Phase One, *Looking Inward*. We will cover the next two phases in proceeding chapters.

When cleaning a closet, what "junk" do you touch first? The junk that falls out when you open it, right?

The words that fell from my head and tumbled out of my mouth were good "junk" to commence the examining. My emotional closet was full and festering.

I said bitterly harsh things —about me. I saw myself as disgusting, as through the eyes of that little boy all those years ago. Every reminder of my weight or my size felt like a crushing blow —a confirmation of my worst thoughts about myself. Even though people had said things to me over the years, no one ever intended them as harshly as I turned them on myself. How had my being overweight become so reprehensible to me? And getting thin become so disproportionately important to me? I might have been willing to club a baby seal if it would make me as thin as a *Victoria's Secret* model.

Instead, I was clubbing *myself* constantly. In a rare moment of objectivity, I noticed that my self-berating routine was not only unhelpful; it was ridiculous. It was time to come to terms with my self-deprecation and toss the emotional toxic waste.

A good place to start on the path to genuine change is by Looking Inward and following these four steps.

1. Explore Your Motives and Desires

Have you ever stepped back and examined your thoughts objectively? What unhelpful thoughts cycle and recycle in your mind? Jot down what comes to your mind. Would you say any of these things to another person? A child? Would Jesus use these words in speaking to you or about you? If the answer is no, ask the Lord for His help in reshaping what's going on in your head, and replace it with the truth of His Word.

As you examine, simply take inventory. Don't start trying to fix anything; just notice what's residing there. This is not a goal-setting exercise. It is an evaluation of your thoughts and desires just as they are. Questions like these may help you identify what's there:

- What drives your desire to lose weight?

- What do you anticipate losing weight would do for you? Your life? (Don't spare the details; be as descriptive as possible. Also, don't judge your thoughts as right or wrong, simply examine what's there.)

- Describe how you've imagined life at your goal weight would be different than your life today.

My visions of being at my goal weight included a few healthy reasons peppered with a litany of irrational ones. For example, I always thought being thin would make me worthy of acceptance. I imagined my life, career, relationships, everything would be radically different at my goal weight. I had built it up as a fantasy in my mind. In doing so, I had also exacerbated my present misery.

In prayer, ask the Lord to help you see your thoughts with His eyes and His wisdom. Describe your struggle to Him in prayer. Cry out if needed. For me, this took many sessions —many prayers, many questions. Many painful things were exposed, including my own sin and pride. Was it fun? No. But it was life-saving and life-giving. Rescue always is.

2. Be Honest

Now that you have explored your motives and desires, the next step is to apply some honesty. Pray for the Lord's direction as you sort through the motives and desires you discovered and wrote down. There are several ways our dishonesty with ourselves may show up.

Do you remember the Samaritan woman Jesus encountered at the well? You can read about her in John 4. She was an outcast in many ways, a racially and socially shunned woman. Jesus knew she had an eventful past. Still, He went out of His way to meet her and to have a tender, patient, and compassionate conversation with her. To the woman's surprise, Jesus didn't condemn her. Instead, He showed her grace and revealed to her that He was the Christ. Her story encouraged me. I was safe to be honest with Him. If there was anyone who could handle the emotional toxic waste I carried around, it was Jesus.

In the safety of His loving presence, examine your heart for untruths you have allowed to pollute your mind and heart. There are three ways you may be harboring untruths: 1) Denial, 2) minimizing the problem, and 3) displacing blame.

As I describe how each one affected me, I invite you to examine your heart for these and any other untruths that may be lurking there.

Denial

Denial was a big obstacle for me. The list was long. One of the biggest issues I was in denial about was how much I ate. I tried to give the impression that I ate like a bird. Too bad it was Big Bird. Another was my intense aversion to the scale. My most feared confrontation in the world was standing on that evil appliance. You would have thought it was waterboarding rather than weighing.

Other common examples of denial might include ignoring health risks, experiencing strained relationships, fostering addictions to salt or sugar, missing ministry or social opportunities, or not seeing the impact habits have on others, especially children. Can you relate? Do any sound familiar?

Examining our own denial isn't an easy step, but it's an important one. But be encouraged. When you bring your emotional obstacles into the light, you and the Lord can work on them together. When you look at them in His light, you'll see they start to lose their power over you. Remember the Samaritan woman and be comforted knowing you are safe to do this in the presence of Jesus.

Minimizing

What's one more cookie? I have already had 6. 10. Whatever. With a finely-honed ability to minimize, I pretended none of my actions were a big deal. One great illustration of minimizing is the old joke, "Other than *that*, Mrs. Lincoln, how did you like the play?" Are you downplaying important indications you ought to face?

I minimized the long-term impact of each impulse I indulged, especially the spiritual impact. I pretended my obsession and self-abuse were nothing. In my mind, I didn't have a problem, and even if I did, it wasn't a big deal. Who was I hurting? Minimizing ensured my appetite got its way without much of a fight. I hadn't even begun to consider what a barrier it was in my relationship with God.

In what ways has "minimizing" your situation and choices impacted you?

Blame

No good self-deception is complete without being able to throw off some blame. Blame is another mind game I used to deflect responsibility like a goalie deflects a torrent of hockey pucks. I was protecting myself from many things, such as the pain of judgment and criticism I expected from others.

I blamed my weight on my "big frame" and my "slow metabolism." Blaming factors outside of my control convinced me my effort was futile. It got me off the hook, or so I thought. All it did was ensure I remained stuck. I used it as permission to console myself with food.

Blaming myself was no better. When thinking, *I'm weak, bad, wrong, hopeless, and unworthy*, I convinced myself the battle was lost, and I need not try.

Blaming anything, anyone, or yourself is useless and destructive. Perhaps that's why the devil uses it. Blaming myself gave me an excuse to try and then quit for any reason or no reason at all.

My three hiding places or strategies were denial, minimizing, and blaming. Exposing them was uncomfortable, like pulling back a bandage to see an infected wound. In hindsight, it's odd that I finally took that step, considering how long, hard, and cleverly I had fought to avoid it. I have no explanation except I knew I was at the end of all my options, and the Lord was at work.

I didn't realize how badly I needed it, or that it was already in process, but God met me where I was. In His presence, I looked inside my heart with honesty and transparency.

He is willing, able, and wants to help. Was I willing to receive His help? What would it cost me? The question takes us to the next step in *Looking Inward.*

3. *Count the Cost*

All decisions require choices. *Wanting* is one thing. *Doing what's required* to obtain something we want is another. When having something means not having another thing, relative desire is tested. Did I really want to be thin as badly as I thought I did? Why was I willing to do anything BUT look honestly at what I was eating? That's when I bumped into it—my wall of unwillingness. I'd go so far, but no further.

That wall protected a stronghold, my "freedom" to eat what I wanted. My food choices were off limits for examination or questioning. Apparently, not even I was supposed to get close to the topic. It was the job of denial, minimizing, and blame to ensure I never confronted myself.

My "freedom" to eat as I pleased (or as pleased me) was so well-protected, no battle to lose weight could penetrate it or outlast it. Even if I was "dieting," I withheld my full commitment to the diet. I reserved the right to say, "I'm done; get the brownies" whenever I felt like it. It was like being engaged knowing you never intended to marry the person because there was someone else. The cost I was feeling of this type of freedom was perpetual misery and shame.

Counting the cost in the presence of God showed me I had a new cost to consider and a new choice to make. It was no longer whether I wanted to be thin. I had to decide whether I wanted to live under the control of my appetite. I also needed to see for the first time that there was a spiritual battle and a spiritual cost to fighting for the wrong team.

I was defeated. *Food and eating had more control over me than I had over them.* Could I change if I wanted to? Did I really want to?

Jesus asked a "counting the cost" question to His followers in Luke 14:31-32. *"What king, going to make war against another king, does not sit down first and consider whether he is able with ten thousand to meet him who comes against him with twenty thousand? And if not, while the other is yet a great way off, he sends a delegation and asks for terms of peace."*

I was fighting a battle I could never win. I was that king making war against a greater King, who happened to be Jesus. What were the terms of peace? I would be wise to learn what they were.

I didn't have what it would take to win the fight against my appetite. I had nearly lost sight of what I was fighting for.

Was the fight to be thin (and all I envisioned went with it) worth all that I had given it? I was fighting the rich rulers fight, the fight to "save" my life. *"For whoever would save his life will lose it, but whoever loses his life for my sake will save it"* (Luke 9:24).

He was inviting me to make peace. Not with food. Not with my weight. But with Him.

4. Realize You Can't Do It Alone

At the beginning of my *"Looking Inward"* journey, I was discouraged. I had all but given up. I had stopped caring about my weight and wasn't even trying to control what I ate. I lost the desire to do anything about it. But God wasn't content to leave me there. I was poised to learn about the transition from *"impossible with man, but possible with God."*

God faithfully and consistently weaves timely resources into my life. I discovered a book by John Piper, *When I Don't Desire God: How to Fight for Joy.*[2] I imagined God looked at me with mercy and said, "I had better spell it out, or she won't get it."

I had never thought about whether I *desired* God, much less whether I desired Him more than anything else. What did I think He meant when He said I should have no other gods before Him, and to love Him with all my heart, soul, mind and strength? I hadn't thought about it enough, nor taken it to heart for what it is: the way God commands me to relate to Him—as *my* God, my creator, and my sovereign Lord.

John Piper's book demonstrated new possibilities of joy and intimacy in a relationship with God that I never considered possible or expected to experience. Until then, my idea of joy was having six-pack abs, while enjoying a steady diet of Haagen Daz.

He wrote, "When a child of God fights for joy in God, God Himself is the one behind that struggle, giving the will and the power to defeat the enemy of joy." God gave me the desire and the power to desire Him more. And more. The more I desired Him, the more my joy in Him increased and the more I sought to meet Him in His word.

When I agreed with God about where I was—*helpless*—and what I needed more than anything—*Him*—things changed. He changed me, slowly. He was doing the impossible in me, just as He had told His disciples about the rich young ruler —*"What is impossible with man is possible with God."*

I finally understood it as clearly as I had ever understood anything: I couldn't overcome my problem alone. My "problem" wasn't even what I thought it was. It wasn't my fat, my weight, or my food. My weight and eating habits were symptoms of the real problem, a deeper stronghold of sin and pride.

I proved to myself I couldn't overcome this exhausting fight through my personal effort or determination. I was at God's mercy, not yet knowing what an incredible place that was to be.

God used the struggle that had overpowered and oppressed me to bring me to *Him*. He wanted to deliver me from all that to Him. He wasn't out to punish me but save me.

Good news: you don't have the power to overcome anything apart from Him. Embracing our powerlessness is the beginning of freedom and healing for followers of Christ. John Piper said, "We are not left to ourselves to sustain the joy of faith. God fights for us and in us." When God fights for us to experience joy and satisfaction in Him, He is showing us how He delivers us from strongholds. He strengthens our affection for Him. As our affection for Him grows, our affections for lesser things weakens.

I know that to be true. The Lord fought for me when I had given up. I knew it was His work because He was changing my heart in ways I couldn't change it, and wouldn't have known to ask or try.

The journey of looking inward may involve some discomfort as you pray through each of the steps. But the Lord is willing to help you lay aside the encumbrances and replace them with the greatest hope of all. Colossians 1:27 reads, *"To them God chose to make known how great among the Gentiles are the riches of the glory of this mystery, which is Christ in you, the hope of glory."*

God has much more for you than losing weight. My weight may have been my biggest concern, but His biggest concern was my heart. He changed me from the inside. While I was marveling at Him and His work, and falling more in love with Him, my relationship with food was changing. How I felt about myself changed. How I perceived what the problem was changed.

Allow yourself to let go of how you've perceived both the problem and the solution. What is possible when you look at all of it in a new way? His way? What could freedom from this stronghold look like for you?

Reflections

Looking Inward *with Him* will help you work through the resistance that has sabotaged you until now. This is the only place to begin the journey. It's not about the food, or the diet, or your weight. The real battle is in your heart. With His grace, mercy, and guidance, you'll see your battle more clearly, and you'll stop wasting your effort on distractions and dead ends. I pray that as you continue through this book, you'll learn how to fight the battle with the power, help, and Biblical weapons God graciously provides.

Next up? *Looking to God.*

Questions

1. As you think about your current health and weight, in what ways have you:

- Engaged in denial about various aspects of your behavior and beliefs?

- Minimized the consequences of your eating habits?

- Blamed others or factors beyond your control?

- Blamed yourself and given up?

2. Now, take a moment to pray through each of these. Ask the Lord about each of them, being comforted that you are safe with Him. Open the door to new openness with Him:

- Lord, why do I do this to myself?
- How does doing this affect my relationship with You?
- Will You help me to see and respond differently in each of these areas, learning what You want me to do instead?

Please take your time working through these studies. They will help you explore the topics in this chapter. As you read the stories of the following people, try to place yourself in each situation in these encounters with Jesus.

The Rich Young Ruler

Read Matthew 19:16-30.

"And behold, a man came up to him, saying, "Teacher, what good deed must I do to have eternal life?" ¹⁷ And he said to him, "Why do you ask me about what is good? There is only one who is good. If you would enter life, keep the commandments." ¹⁸ He said to him, "Which ones?" And Jesus said, "You shall not murder, You shall not commit adultery, You shall not steal, You shall not bear false witness, ¹⁹ Honor your father and mother, and, You shall love your neighbor as yourself." ²⁰ The young man said to him, "All these I have kept. What do I still lack?" ²¹ Jesus said to him, "If you would be perfect, go, sell what you possess and give to the poor, and you will have treasure in heaven; and come, follow me." ²² When the young man heard this he went away sorrowful, for he had great possessions.

²³ And Jesus said to his disciples, "Truly, I say to you, only with difficulty will a rich person enter the kingdom of heaven. ²⁴ Again I tell you, it is easier for a camel to go through the eye of a needle than for a rich person to enter the kingdom of God." ²⁵ When the disciples heard this, they were greatly astonished, saying, "Who then can be saved?" ²⁶ But Jesus looked at them and said, "With man this is impossible, but with God all things are possible." ²⁷ Then Peter said in reply, "See, we have left everything and followed you. What then will we have?" ²⁸ Jesus said to them, "Truly, I say to you, in the new world, when the Son of Man will sit on his glorious throne, you who have followed me will also sit on twelve thrones, judging the twelve tribes of Israel. ²⁹ And everyone who has left houses or brothers or sisters or father or mother or children or lands, for my name's sake, will receive a hundredfold and will inherit eternal life. ³⁰ But many who are first will be last, and the last first.

1. What answer was the rich young ruler expecting from Jesus?

2. Pretend you are the rich young ruler. Describe what you are thinking and feeling as you hear Jesus' answer.

3. What things (or beliefs) in your life are so much a part of you that they would be hard to leave behind to follow Jesus? (Take heart, everyone struggles with this. But not many press on for Jesus' help to move forward!)

4. What hope does Jesus give the disciples? (Hint: read verse 28-29)

5. Describe the young man's dilemma in your own words. In what way can you relate to him?

6. Write out to the Lord what you've learned from Him in this passage:

The Woman at the Well

Read John 4:16-30.

Jesus said to her, "Go, call your husband, and come here." [17] The woman answered him, "I have no husband." Jesus said to her, "You are right in saying, 'I have no husband'; [18] for you have had five husbands, and the one you now have is not your husband. What you have said is true." [19] The woman said to him, "Sir, I perceive that you are a prophet. [20] Our fathers worshiped on this mountain, but you say that in Jerusalem is the place where people ought to worship." [21] Jesus said to her, "Woman, believe me, the hour is coming when neither on this mountain nor in Jerusalem will you worship the Father. [22] You worship what you do not know; we worship what we know, for salvation is from the Jews. [23] But the hour is coming, and is now here, when the true worshipers will worship the Father in spirit and truth, for the Father is seeking such people to worship him. [24] God is spirit, and those who worship him must worship in spirit and truth." [25] The woman said to him, "I know that Messiah is coming (he who is called Christ). When he comes, he will tell us all things." [26] Jesus said to her, "I who speak to you am he."

[27] Just then his disciples came back. They marveled that he was talking with a woman, but no one said, "What do you seek?" or, "Why are you talking with her?" [28] So the woman left her water jar and went away into town and said to the people, [29] "Come, see a man who told me all that I ever did. Can this be the Christ?" [30] They went out of the town and were coming to him.

1. Imagine going about your business one day and encountering a stranger that turned out to be Jesus. What might Jesus see in your life?

2. As He was with the Samaritan woman, Jesus is fully aware of *everything we ever did*. How does that make you feel?

3. Reflect on your eating habits and your relationship with food. Since Jesus knows even before you explain, how might you ask Him to help you?

4. How willing do you think He is to help you?

5. How comfortable are you talking to Jesus about this area of struggle?

6. Take a moment and tell Him everything you are thinking and feeling about it. Write it out:

The Paralytic by the Pool

Read John 5:2-9.

Now there is in Jerusalem by the Sheep Gate a pool, in Aramaic called Bethesda, which has five roofed colonnades. ³ In these lay a multitude of invalids—blind, lame, and paralyzed. ⁵ One man was there who had been an invalid for thirty-eight years. ⁶ When Jesus saw him lying there and knew that he had already been there a long time, he said to him, "Do you want to be healed?" ⁷ The sick man answered him, "Sir, I have no one to put me into the pool when the water is stirred up, and while I am going another steps down before me." ⁸ Jesus said to him, "Get up, take up your bed, and walk." ⁹ And at once the man was healed, and he took up his bed and walked.

1. What did Jesus ask the paralytic? How did the paralytic respond?

2. Place yourself in the paralytic's circumstances, but your "paralysis" is your weight. Do you have a pre-conceived notion about how He should heal you? What might you be saying to Jesus?

3. Jesus asked the paralytic to do something different than the paralytic thought needed to be done. What was it?

4. How have your preconceived notions prevented you from hearing Jesus? What will you do with those notions?

Zacchaeus

Read Luke 19:1-10.

He entered Jericho and was passing through. ² And behold, there was a man named Zacchaeus. He was a chief tax collector and was rich.³ And he was seeking to see who Jesus was, but on account of the crowd he could not, because he was small in stature. ⁴ So he ran on ahead and climbed up into a sycamore tree to see him, for he was about to pass that way. ⁵ And when Jesus came to the place, he looked up and said to him, "Zacchaeus, hurry and come down, for I must stay at your house today." ⁶ So he hurried and came down and received him joyfully. ⁷ And when they saw it, they all grumbled, "He has gone in to be the guest of a man who is a sinner." ⁸ And Zacchaeus stood and said to the Lord, "Behold, Lord, the half of my goods I give to the poor. And if I have defrauded anyone of anything, I restore it fourfold." ⁹ And Jesus said to him, "Today salvation has come to this house, since he also is a son of Abraham. ¹⁰ For the Son of Man came to seek and to save the lost."

1. Describe what Zacchaeus' was doing in anticipation of Jesus.

2. What did Zacchaeus do after meeting Jesus?

3. In what ways was Zacchaeus' response to Jesus different from the rich ruler's response?

4. Do you identify more with Zacchaeus or the rich young ruler? Why?

5. Look up Matthew 19: 23-26. How does Zacchaeus illustrate what Jesus said? Describe how this gives you hope:

Peter

Read Matthew 26:30-35, 69-75.

And when they had sung a hymn, they went out to the Mount of Olives. ³¹ Then Jesus said to them, "You will all fall away because of me this night. For it is written, 'I will strike the shepherd, and the sheep of the flock will be scattered.' ³² But after I am raised up, I will go before you to Galilee." ³³ Peter answered him, "Though they all fall away because of you, I will never fall away." ³⁴ Jesus said to him, "Truly, I tell you, this very night, before the rooster crows, you will deny me three times." ³⁵ Peter said to him, "Even if I must die with you, I will not deny you!" And all the disciples said the same.

⁶⁹ Now Peter was sitting outside in the courtyard. And a servant girl came up to him and said, "You also were with Jesus the Galilean." ⁷⁰ But he denied it before them all, saying, "I do not know what you mean." ⁷¹ And when he went out to the entrance, another servant girl saw him, and she said to the bystanders, "This man was with Jesus of Nazareth." ⁷² And again he denied it with an oath: "I do not know the man." ⁷³ After a little while the bystanders came up and said to Peter, "Certainly you too are one of them, for your accent betrays you." ⁷⁴ Then he began to invoke a curse on himself and to swear, "I do not know the man." And immediately the rooster crowed. ⁷⁵ And Peter remembered the saying of Jesus, "Before the rooster crows, you will deny me three times." And he went out and wept bitterly.

1. How confident was Peter in what he said in verse 33? What was his confidence based on?

2. Why do you think Peter unable to understand and accept Jesus' forewarning?

3. How confident are you in your own personal capacity for the long-term change of losing weight ?

4. Although Peter experienced this and other failures in his walk with Jesus, he was among the closest of Jesus' disciples. He grew to become an Apostle and leader in the building of the Christian Church. Describe how Peter's growth gives you hope in your own relationship with Christ:

Chapter Four:
Who's your Daddy?

My dad was an attorney and a bit of a workaholic. To me, he was like Atticus Finch, the main character in *To Kill a Mockingbird*. He was a Southern gentleman: kind, wise, unpretentious, and generous. People often brought him gifts for the work he did for them.

As much as I respected admired him, my dad and I weren't close during my childhood. We didn't spend much time together. He seemed distant. I knew he cared about me, provided well for me, and had high hopes and standards for me. I wanted to please him and live up to those standards. But I didn't really know him. I wasn't quite sure if I wanted to be close to him, or if he wanted to be close to me. In a way, distance was easier. Emotions were awkward, even painful. I was happy *not* to feel them.

Since my dad passed away, I've reflected on my relationship with him and noticed my similar thoughts about God. He was my Heavenly Father, but to me, He too was distant and unknowable, and that was "normal." It felt normal to admire Him from afar and not seek emotional closeness. I figured He was busy with the big stuff, like gravity, air traffic control for the galaxies, and, of course, people who were way worse off than I was. My job? Just to live, refrain from doing anything overtly reprehensible, and occasionally perform a random act of kindness. I never questioned my flawed theology. I didn't know that more was possible. Distance was easier with my heavenly Father as it had been with my earthly father.

"Distant" does not describe the kind of relationship God desires with His children. *I* didn't know I needed more of Him, but *He* did.

My weight contributed to the distance between my earthly father and me. I knew my weight displeased him. It's no surprise that I wanted to avoid God as well when it came to my weight. But there came a time when was my frustration boiled over into crying out for Him.

Looking to God is the second phase of the Spiritual Model of Change. It's a necessary progression from *Looking Inward,* adding a much-needed grander perspective to our myopia.

In his book *Crazy Love*, Francis Chan wrote, "If my mind is the size of a soda can and God is the size of all the oceans, it would be stupid for me to say He is only the small amount of water I can scoop into my little can. God is so much bigger, so far beyond our time-encased, air-food-sleep-dependent lives."[3]

As you think about how you relate to God, take a moment to pray that He will give you a growing hunger to know Him, and to never be satisfied with only what you know right now. Have your thoughts and feelings limited your expectations and hopes in God? Mine did until He showed me otherwise.

Looking to God

Turning to God with my thoughts and feelings about my weight was awkward. Even painful. Taking small steps helped tremendously. These small steps below will guide you through *Looking to God*, the next phase in the Spiritual Model of Change.

Let's look at each of the four steps: **Believe, Trust, Honor, and Offer.**

1. Believe from the Heart

The word *believe* used to confuse me, especially as it related to believing in Jesus. James 2:19 says, *"You believe that God is one; you do well. Even the demons believe—and shudder!"* That phrase made *me* shudder and question myself about how I believed. Did I believe in God the same way the demons believe Jesus is God, but reject His Lordship and refuse to follow Him? Why was I unsettled over the word *believe*?

I thought about the rich young ruler. He met Jesus face to face and walked away. Then, I thought about Zacchaeus and his encounter with Jesus. It was quite a contrast. Let's examine it together.

Reading his story in Luke 19:1-10, did you notice Zacchaeus reacted differently to Jesus from the start? Zacchaeus ran to catch a glimpse of Jesus, and scurried up a tree to get a better view. Why was he so eager? Jesus saw him and shared a meal with him, of all people, the chief tax collector. Imagine if Jesus came to your town and dined with the person who was most widely despised. But this outcast (albeit rich) tax official was about to be transformed by Jesus. A rich man? Saved? Didn't Jesus just say that was impossible? What was different about Zacchaeus?

When Zacchaeus addressed Jesus, he called him *Lord*, unlike the rich young ruler who had addressed Jesus as "Teacher." Zacchaeus believed Jesus was the Son of God. Then, Zacchaeus did something else that differed from the rich ruler. In his response to Jesus, Zacchaeus declared,

"Behold, Lord, the half of my goods I give to the poor. And if I have defrauded anyone of anything, I restore it fourfold" (Luke 19:8).

Jesus hadn't said anything to him about his money or asked for such a gesture from him. Why did the two rich men respond so differently?

Notice the way they *believed* in Jesus. One rich man saw Jesus as a teacher. The other rich man believed Jesus was the Son of God. Zacchaeus' actions reflected that he believed Jesus to be far greater than his life and possessions. No, he didn't have to stop and calculate. On the contrary, the rich ruler's response reflected that his own life, as it was, had great value to him. He wasn't expecting to have to choose between the life he lived now and eternal life.

Yes, Jesus had said to the disciples that it was difficult for a rich man to enter heaven. However, He also said, *"what is impossible with man is possible with God"* (Luke 18:27). I love the way Jesus demonstrated through Zacchaeus so specifically what God makes possible in the heart of "impossible" people—people who believe in who Jesus is, not who they wish Jesus was, or who they limit Him to in their minds.

These incidents illustrate what Jesus said in Matthew 16:25. *"For whoever would save his life will lose it, but whoever loses his life for my sake will find it."* The rich ruler chose to save his earthly life at the cost of eternal life in Christ. Zacchaeus recognized the incomparable worth of Jesus, and his perception of the value of his own life and possessions lost its hold on him.

When I looked inward at my heart, I noticed a long history of thinking like the rich young ruler. Why didn't I respond to Jesus the way Zacchaeus had? In my spirit, I knew I needed help with my *unbelief.*

My typical impulse is to immediately look for what to *do*. If something needs fixing, I am like Quick Draw McGraw with an action plan. But Zacchaeus was not transformed by what he *did;* he was transformed by *whom* he believed.

What was lacking in my belief about Jesus, causing me to more resembled the rich young ruler than Zacchaeus?

What does my belief in Jesus as the Son of God have to do with my weight problem? Perhaps the connection would be clearer if you imagine that these two men, rather than being rich, were addicted to food. One was not willing to leave his "idol." The other's encounter with Jesus freed him from his idol to take hold of something he recognized was incomparably better.

I hadn't experienced a Zacchaeus-like transformation that freed me from this lifelong battle, my relationship with food, and all the emotional baggage tied up in it. Something supernatural happened in Zacchaeus' heart. Whatever it was, I needed it. It wasn't salad, jumping jacks, diet pills, or liposuction. I had tried all those, just as the rich young ruler had done his best to keep the Mosaic Law. He and I both hoped we would be able to obtain what we most wanted with our own efforts without giving up what we already had. We would do exactly what was required to have what we most wanted. Well, except one thing—let it go to follow Jesus.

My comparison of these two rich men left me with questions and no one to ask for answers, except God. He had answered me already, but I had avoided turning to Him. Instead, I insisted on trying everything else I knew to do. I wanted it to work *my* way, on *my* terms. But my way didn't work. It was an endless, frustrating waste of time. I was helpless. When I finally looked to Him, I saw how stubborn I was, not listening and trying to negotiate a good deal for myself. I recognized I was in a power struggle I couldn't win. And I was fighting for something worthless (relative to the worth of Jesus) at the cost of my soul. I wanted Jesus' help. But I didn't want Jesus Himself. I didn't want His authority over me. It occurred to me, *That's probably similar to what the demons want.* And that's concerning.

What do you believe about Jesus? How do you feel about being honest with God and yourself about your weight and relationship with food? Have you, like me, tried to hide this area of your life from Him? Have you insisted on doing things *your* way? Whether you feel apprehensive or wide open, God meets you where you are; simply reach out to Him.

I once heard preacher Adrian Rogers say, "God loves you right where you are, but He loves you too much to leave you there." Ask the Lord to help you believe in Him for who He is. As your belief deepens, you'll see the "why," the "what," and the "how" of your struggle to lose weight in a new light, in His light. You'll realize it's not about the food, the diet, or even your weight any more than it was about the rich ruler's riches. Believing in Jesus as Lord leads to the next step: trusting.

2. Shift Your Trust

Your deepening belief prepares the way for the next step. If belief is high school, trust is college. Trust is a step of faith based on belief. Trust is acting on what we believe but can't yet see. Everyone tends to resist following God when it involves something seemingly impossible or undesirable. Embracing the reality that we are not in control is a test of our trust, our willingness to entrust ourselves to Him.

All my life, I would have said I trusted God. But, my trust was untested. I avoided situations that tested my trust, or made me vulnerable, needing to lean on God.

Throughout Scripture, the Lord intentionally leads His children into situations where He tests them. He does the same for us now, and it's for our good. Granted, those opportunities are rarely fun, and we wouldn't choose them for ourselves. But tests are God's way of showing us where we are and helping us grow. What if your struggle with your weight is a test of your faith and an opportunity to grow in Him?

Have you known people who have endured hardship, yet wouldn't trade what God taught them for an easier time? They would never have gained spiritually what God gave them had they remained untested in safety or comfort.

God has a bigger purpose for developing our trust. Yes, He knows we need to trust Him, but He also intends to amplify our trust in Him for the greater good of His Kingdom. His design is for more than our personal benefit. His Word confirms this in Romans 8:28-29. *"And we know that for those who love God all things work together for good, for those who are called according to his purpose. ²⁹ For those whom he foreknew he also predestined to be conformed to the image of his Son, in order that he might be the firstborn among many brothers."* The Lord tests us to develop Christ in us, conforming us to His image.

Which has more value, reaching an idealized size or weight, or being conformed to the image of Christ? What if the testing you've experienced in the battle with your weight has the outcome of molding you into the likeness of Christ?

Do you trust God enough to move forward, through occasional discomfort? What if you knew He would bring you victory over your challenges through His work in you? What if doing so would draw you closer to God than ever before and equip you to serve Him more effectively?

Real spiritual change takes time and requires endurance. While God is working, we are also working with Him. We must leave old comfortable routines behind and establish new ones. Change has a messy middle part between where you are and where you are headed. During the transition, new behaviors don't quite fit yet. They feel awkward. You may occasionally long for your old habits, routines, and comforts. It's normal. It's helpful to realize the work of change is not simply leaving behind the habits that hold you back. You will be moving forward with a new perspective and learning how to seek the Lord to heal and satisfy you in the areas you've been enslaved.

Ask the Lord to help you trust Him. Look for each opportunity to choose Him rather than the choice that keeps you stuck in your current routine. Letting a craving go unfilled is only uncomfortable temporarily. Each time you do it, He is strengthening you.

Fully trusting God requires endurance. Our old habits have offered us pleasure on demand. The breakup may feel hard. Why? Because God's reward is spiritual. Foregoing a craving is making a declaration: "I'm willing to say no to my desires and yes to God, and therefore, I'm willing to suffer through a craving rather than indulge it."

When the pleasure, relief, and comforts of food are absent, our inner condition is exposed: dissatisfaction, stress, and discomfort. If we are unprepared, we can't endure the messy place for very long. Without shifting our trust to God, we won't endure long enough to see *how* God addresses our raw feelings, much less allow Him to do so. It's not only possible but necessary to lean into trusting God. In fact, the word "trust" means to "lean." We can lean on God and know that He will support us. You can *trust* Him to be with you in each decision you make. He is with you even in the discomfort of it.

The comfort God gives is real, but it is different from the comfort our old habits bring. God's comfort felt different than eating made me feel. God's comfort won't feel like the immediate gratification of your favorite foods. And you may still experience those cravings, but they will pass and diminish as you let them go unfulfilled.

How do you imagine God will comfort you? How will you experience it? Can He comfort you spiritually, while still allowing you to feel physical or emotional discomfort? What will you do when the new trust you are developing toward God requires you to endure and address feelings you were stifling with food? Entrust yourself to Him, to His Word, and to prayer. Allow yourself to feel the discomfort, and thank Him for revealing the way your flesh wants to overtake you. When you feel that struggle take note, that is the enemy you are fighting against so that you will have more of Christ in you.

If you have ever been ill and had someone care for you, you know they cannot take away the sickness or suffering, but there is tremendous comfort in them coming alongside you. Welcome God to come alongside you in the challenge of change, and know you will grow closer to Him each time you lean on Him and allow yourself to endure the absence of old comforts. You'll see that His comfort is real and far deeper, more lasting and better than any momentary distraction food can offer. His comfort will not only sustain you in the messy middle but see you through it.

3. Honor Whose You Are

Imagine the Apostle Paul alive today. What would he write to the church in America? It might be similar to the letter he wrote to the Corinthians. Many problems had arisen in the church. One of the sins Paul called out was sexual immorality. But their sin exposed an assumption they made about their bodies. They assumed their bodies were their own to do with as they pleased.

In I Corinthians 6:19-21, Paul wrote, *"Or do you not know that your body is a temple of the Holy Spirit within you, whom you have from God? You are not your own, for you were bought with a price. So glorify God in your body."* Have you ever reflected on that verse in view of your relationship with food?

As Christians, we face all kinds of physical temptations, including the temptation to overeat. When Paul spoke of glorifying God in our bodies, he was saying we must live in a way that honors God and reflects we know what He did when He saved us. We became His. Our ownership changed, literally.

Christ's death on my behalf purchased me from another owner: sin and death. I didn't immediately grasp what that meant for me. God's forgiveness is unlike human forgiveness. It accomplishes something supernatural, eternal. I was forgiven, but was I released back to the wild with a blank check to do what I want, even to sin? *If I am forgiven*, in such a transcendent way, I wondered, *does it matter if I overeat, or for that matter, smoke, drink, take drugs, fornicate, or watch porn?* I envisioned Bill Murray in the movie *Groundhog Day*, gorging himself and chain smoking. Every day was a do-over and nothing he had done the day before mattered. I wouldn't have said it out loud, but I lived as though my sin and my sinning no longer mattered. How had I gotten that impression about salvation? What was I missing?

In Galatians 5:13 and in Romans 6:1, Paul answered a similar question. There was a group of new believers in Christ who thought the more they sinned, the more they received of God's grace. They apparently thought, "Let's sin more and make it rain grace up in here." They were mistaken, as was I.

Imagine you started a fire in your house by smoking in bed. A fireman rescued you, losing his life in the process. Then, not long after, you repeated the incident—smoking, falling asleep, starting a fire. Another fireman's life was lost rescuing you. Would it be appropriate for you to say, "I should smoke in bed more because I'm glorifying the bravery of the fire department?" To do so would be a failure to grasp the seriousness of your actions and the value of lives of your rescuers.

I was doing the same thing toward God. I underestimated the depth of my sin and that my sin, like all sin, was against God Himself. I also minimized the price He paid to save me. I was dishonoring God

"For you were called to freedom, brothers. Only do not use your freedom as an opportunity for the flesh, but through love, serve one another" (Galatians 5:13). My salvation was a clean slate in terms of my sin, but not a blank check to go on sinning. To do so is an affront to God Himself.

In the book, *Jesus Among Other Gods*, author Ravi Zacharias explains the uniqueness of God's indwelling of us. "The Christian does not go to the temple to worship. The Christian takes the temple with him or her. Jesus lifts us beyond the building and pays the human body the highest compliment by making it His dwelling place, the place where He meets us. Even today, He would overturn the tables of those who make it a marketplace for their own lust, greed, and wealth."

I asked myself, *How different would my decisions look if I genuinely believed God dwells in me? If I am His temple, holy, set apart, purchased with the sacrifice of Christ, so that He can dwell in me, how should that affect what I do, say, feel, think, and live?* At the time I first asked myself these questions, I didn't know the answer. I only knew my life ought to look quite different than it did.

How about you? Do you genuinely believe God dwells in you? If so, are your choices honoring God? I know that may be an uncomfortable question, but it's an important question to explore in prayer. It will help you connect your daily choices and your relationship with the Lord. You live in the body He purchased with His blood and where He dwells. Honoring the One who made, died for, and now dwells in us means that we must live according to this truth.

4. Offer Yourself to Him

The fourth step in *Looking to God* is to offer yourself to Him. In my life, I've spent more years misunderstanding genuine faith than I've spent living it out. I was going through the motions and trying to "do it right." I had a loosely defined idea of what a Christian should and shouldn't do. I gave myself undue credit for meaning well, trying hard, and being a "good enough" person. I was pleased with myself for following this standard. What more could I do? I didn't think about whether I was surrendered to the Lord. I assumed I was, but based on what? I have no idea. If I was pleased with myself, God probably was too, right? Scripture didn't support my assumption.

Romans 12:1 reads, *"I appeal to you therefore, brothers, by the mercies of God, to present your bodies as a living sacrifice, holy and acceptable to God, which is your spiritual worship."* I must have read this verse hundreds of times, but did I ever ponder what it required of me? Or that I had no idea how to respond in obedience?

Offering myself to God has been a wrestling match. Surrendering to the Lord isn't easy, nor has it come naturally. It calls upon me to make an effort. But doing what? The best answer I could find to help me understand was in Philippians 2:12-13. Paul says, *"Therefore, my beloved, as you have always obeyed, so now, not only as in my presence but much more in my absence, work out your own salvation with fear and trembling, for it is God who works in you, both to will and to work for his good pleasure."*

God works in me as I surrender and cooperate with His work in me. Offering myself to God is none of the following:

- natural.
- a one-time thing.
- a polite suggestion on His part.

Offering yourself to God is a pivotal step in your life as a follower of Christ. In a surrendered life, you'll discover His power to overcome what besets or encumbers you. Once we make the decision to give our lives to Him, He helps us grow in the ability to offer ourselves to Him.

In the next chapter, we'll discuss the way God involves other people on this journey. *Looking to Community* is the final phase in the Spiritual Model of Change.

Reflections

Can you envision yourself moving through the process of Believing, Trusting, Honoring, and Offering? Consider each a stepping stone to placing yourself in God's hands. With each step, we grow more accepting of this truth: None of us can achieve freedom on our own. By *Looking to God*, we do not gain "the upper hand." Instead, we gain God's *mighty* hand, which helps us overcome strongholds that have us beat.

Questions

This is a longer Questions section, so you may want to move through each step (Believing, Trusting, Honoring, Offering) in individual sessions. Don't push yourself to rush through these steps, but take the time to think through and absorb each one.

Step 1: Believing
Read Mark 9:14-29.

And when they came to the disciples, they saw a great crowd around them, and scribes arguing with them. 15 And immediately all the crowd, when they saw him, were greatly amazed and ran up to him and greeted him. 16 And he asked them, "What are you arguing about with them?"

17 And someone from the crowd answered him, "Teacher, I brought my son to you, for he has a spirit that makes him mute. 18 And whenever it seizes him, it throws him down, and he foams and grinds his teeth and becomes rigid. So I asked your disciples to cast it out, and they were not able."

19 And he answered them, "O faithless generation, how long am I to be with you? How long am I to bear with you? Bring him to me." 20 And they brought the boy to him. And when the spirit saw him, immediately it convulsed the boy, and he fell on the ground and rolled about, foaming at the mouth. 21 And Jesus asked his father, "How long has this been happening to him?" And he said, "From childhood. 22 And it has often cast him into fire and into water, to destroy him. But if you can do anything, have compassion on us and help us."

23 And Jesus said to him, "'If you can'! All things are possible for one who believes." 24 Immediately the father of the child cried out[a] and said, "I believe; help my unbelief!" 25 And when Jesus saw that a crowd came running together, he rebuked the unclean spirit, saying to it, "You mute and deaf spirit, I command you, come out of him and never enter him again." ²⁶ *And after crying out and convulsing him terribly, it came out, and the boy was like a corpse, so that most of them said, "He is dead."*

²⁷ *But Jesus took him by the hand and lifted him up, and he arose.* ²⁸ *And when he had entered the house, his disciples asked him privately, "Why could we not cast it out?"* ²⁹ *And he said to them, "This kind cannot be driven out by anything but prayer."*

1. What made it difficult for the father to believe that Jesus could help his son?

2. What emotions might the father have been feeling?

3. As it relates to losing weight, have you ever felt like the father of the boy might have felt? How so?

4. When we bring our most difficult battles to Jesus, it's helpful to see that we are turning to God Himself. Describe how this is different than all the other things you have tried:

5. Write out what Jesus asked the man in verse 21.

6. How did the man answer?

7. What did Jesus say?

8. Why do you think Jesus said what He said to the man, rather than simply healing the man's son?

9. Who heard Jesus say what He said?

10. Imagine you were coming to Jesus with the same emotions and frustrations as the man, but it is about your weight. Write out what you would say to Him.

11. When Jesus asks you, "How long has this been happening?"—what would you say?

12. Based on what Jesus did for the man and his son, how does that influence what you think Jesus could do for you?

13. What is required on your part?

14. What kind of help did the man ask for?

15. Do you need the same kind of help from Jesus?

16. Write out your prayer to Him.

Step 2: Trusting

Read Matthew 14:22-33.

Immediately he made the disciples get into the boat and go before him to the other side, while he dismissed the crowds. 23 And after he had dismissed the crowds, he went up on the mountain by himself to pray. When evening came, he was there alone, 24 but the boat by this time was a long way from the land, beaten by the waves, for the wind was against them. 25 And in the fourth watch of the night he came to them, walking on the sea. 26 But when the disciples saw him walking on the sea, they were terrified, and said, "It is a ghost!" and they cried out in fear. 27 But immediately Jesus spoke to them, saying, "Take heart; it is I. Do not be afraid."

28 And Peter answered him, "Lord, if it is you, command me to come to you on the water." 29 He said, "Come." So Peter got out of the boat and walked on the water and came to Jesus. 30 But when he saw the wind, he was afraid, and beginning to sink he cried out, "Lord, save me." 31 Jesus immediately reached out his hand and took hold of him, saying to him, "O you of little faith, why did you doubt?" 32 And when they got into the boat, the wind ceased. 33 And those in the boat worshiped him, saying, "Truly you are the Son of God."

1. When Jesus sent the disciples across the sea, did the disciples know there was a storm ahead?

2. Jesus knew He was sending them into a storm – why do you think He did it anyway?

3. Imagine the scene. Verse 25 revealed it was the 4th watch of the night. The storm had these men, some of them seasoned fishermen, embattled. How did they first react when they saw Jesus? (See verse 26.)

4. What are some reasons why they may have reacted that way?

5. What did Jesus say?

6. What exactly did Peter say?

7. What word did Peter use that the father of the demon-possessed boy also used?

8. Whose idea was it for Peter to walk on the water?

9. Why do you think Jesus answered Peter's request?

10. Describe step by step what happened in verse 29 and 30.

11. What did Jesus do?

12. What did Jesus say?

13. What happened to the storm?

14. How did the men react?

15. Reflect for a moment about everything the disciples learned about Jesus from this incident that they didn't know about Him before it happened. List everything you can think of.

16. If Jesus has power over diseases, demons, and nature, what power does He have over your strongholds?

17. What does Jesus teach us in circumstances like storms and life's difficulties?

18. In what ways does this story demonstrate the difference between believing and trusting?

Step 3: Honoring

Read 1 Corinthians 6:12-20. **Note:** Paul is specifically addressing sexual immorality in this passage. Nevertheless, his reasoning is helpful in addressing all of our behaviors that stand in the way of our right conduct before God.

"All things are lawful for me," but not all things are helpful. "All things are lawful for me," but I will not be dominated by anything. [13] "Food is meant for the stomach and the stomach for food"—and God will destroy both one and the other. The body is not meant for sexual immorality, but for the Lord, and the Lord for the body. [14] And God raised the Lord and will also raise us up by his power. [15] Do you not know that your bodies are members of Christ? Shall I then take the members of Christ and make them members of a prostitute? Never! [16] Or do you not know that he who is joined to a prostitute becomes one body with her? For, as it is written, "The two will become one flesh." [17] But he who is joined to the Lord becomes one spirit with him. [18] Flee from sexual immorality. Every other sin a person commits is outside the body, but the sexually immoral person sins against his own body. [19] Or do you not know that your body is a temple of the Holy Spirit within you, whom you have from God? You are not your own, [20] for you were bought with a price. So glorify God in your body.

1. In verse 12, Paul is apparently quoting and responding to an argument that someone had made to justify their bad behavior. What self-justifying argument was made in verse 12?

2. What were Paul's two replies to this argument in verse 12?

3. What do you think Paul meant by each of these two arguments?

4. How can an area of false freedom come to "master" us?

5. In verses 13 and 14, Paul is not only saying what the body is not for but what it is for. Write out what Paul says the body is for in verse 13.

6. Write out verse 14.

7. What does it mean that we are raised up by His power?

8. Read the first part of verse 15. How does knowing that your body is a member of Christ influence your perception of what you do every day? Specifically, what implications does it have on how you approach eating?

9. Having read and reflected on the verses leading up to verses 19 and 20, write out what it means to you that your body is the dwelling place of the Holy Spirit?

10. What does it mean *to you* that you have been bought with a price?

11. It can be daunting to realize that our bodies are not ours to do with as we please. How do you feel about this right now?

12. Write out a prayer to the Lord describing to Him what you have just learned:

13. What help would you like to ask Him for?

Step 4: Offering
Read Romans 12:1-2.

I appeal to you therefore, brothers, by the mercies of God, to present your bodies as a living sacrifice, holy and acceptable to God, which is your spiritual worship. ² Do not be conformed to this world, but be transformed by the renewal of your mind, that by testing you may discern what is the will of God, what is good and acceptable and perfect.

These verses are quite familiar to many people. Verse 1 begins with "Therefore" and is the culmination of some very heavy-duty, awesome, and incredible exhortation on the part of the Apostle Paul.

Offering our bodies as a living sacrifice is no small thing. It is not as though we can respond to it with "Yep, got it, I'll get right on that." It is difficult to grasp what it really means, especially apart from the Holy Spirit opening our eyes and hearts to reveal what it means in our own lives, right where we are.

1. What do you think it means to "not be conformed to this world"?

2. According to this verse, what is the outcome of renewing our minds?

3. What does Paul mean when he says, "that by testing we may discern what is the will of God?"

4. How does Paul describe the will of God in the phrase that follows?

5. Ask the Lord to help you understand what it means to offer your body as a living sacrifice.

6. How important is it that you understand what it means? Be sure to express why it is important to you personally.

Chapter Five:
Help!

Recall the first two phases of the Spiritual Model of Change, *Looking Inward* and *Looking to God*. Both phases encourage spiritual searching, prayer, and reflection. This is "heart work." You can do in peace, quiet, and privacy. The work is critical to forming the spiritual foundation for the actions you will be taking in your weight loss journey. The rest of the journey doesn't happen when you're alone.

The final phase of the Spiritual Model of Change is *Looking to Community*. This component is perhaps the most overlooked and underestimated part of long-term change. How do the people in your life affect you? How will they respond to your weight loss efforts?

Losing weight isn't a solo sport like tennis, where winning or losing depends only on you. Your weight loss journey affects other people, and they affect you. This adds unpredictability. Think rugby; some will help you score while others will knock you down and try to take the ball from you, figuratively speaking. Because your weight journey happens amidst other humans from start to finish, it is important to plan accordingly to ensure your "team" is aligned with you, and you are sensitive to the ways your life affects them.

We all need the help of others in our lives, especially when overcoming the obstacles we face. In this chapter, we'll discuss the necessary steps to ensure your community is aligned and prepared to help you reach your destination. First, it is necessary to clarify what the word "help" means and to identify the types of help and support you're going to need.

Unhelpful Help

Not all help is helpful. Sometimes, the best intentions of those closest to you can go awry. Here's a true story (confession)that illustrates unhelpful help.

The room was dark except for the harsh fluorescent lights over Daddy's head. The clock said 2:37 a.m. A piercing beep made me jump nervously, like a shell-shocked soldier. His IV line was blocked again. Daddy had suffered a stroke five days earlier. In this moment, he had just been returned to his room after a short surgical procedure to give him a pacemaker.

In his usual style, he sat wide awake, almost chipper. He acted as though nothing unusual was going on, even though moments ago, he had been cut open to have a battery-operated object placed in his chest and plugged into his beating heart.

The stern-looking night nurse had been marching in and out to silence the loud beeping. She was about as gentle as a tire iron. She reminded me of Nurse Ratched from the novel-turned-movie, *One Flew Over the Cuckoo's Nest*.

She should work in a prison, not a hospital, I thought to myself. I found her demeanor intimidating and her lack of warmth toward my father annoying. Still, I had no desire to tangle with her.

My annoyance was growing. No one seemed to be in any big rush to ease Daddy's suffering. He hadn't eaten for five days, while countless specialists took turns assessing his condition. All that time, the doctor's orders were "nil per os" or "NPO,, which means, "May the wrath of Heaven come down on you if you give this patient anything to eat or drink." This instruction had faded from my awareness as I asked Daddy if he was hungry. He nodded. I was not surprised. My inner voice spoke up, *What does it take to get a man some food in this joint?* It was time to take matters into my own hands.

There was nothing to eat at the hospital at 2:37 a.m. except vending machine fare. Locating one down the hall, I assessed the array of options. For a reason I cannot explain, I thought the ham sandwich looked like a good choice for Daddy. Row G, Number 3. Yes, I purchased a ham sandwich from a vending machine—something I had never considered doing before, nor since, under any circumstance.

I toted the sandwich back to the room like a coonhound with its quarry. I handed it to Daddy. He unwrapped it and bit into it with gusto, just like a man who hadn't eaten in five days. I felt delighted! I had brought long-overdue relief to my long-suffering dad.

A few bites later, his bending arm made the IV line clog, and the machine began beeping again. Nurse Ratched came right away and saw Daddy noshing on the best pork and white bread $1.25 could buy. Words cannot describe her reaction, but let's just say I was tempted to call an exorcist. She was aghast at the sight of a post-op patient eating a ham sandwich!

Nurse Ratched mustered great restraint to refrain from choking me with the catheter tubing she was holding. Spittle flew out of her mouth as she described the risk I had placed Daddy in.

After recovering from her humiliating tongue-lashing, reality hit me. I could have seriously harmed him. In my impulsive need to help—to do anything to relieve just a little of Daddy's suffering—I could have harmed him. Praise the Lord that Daddy had no ill effects from the ham sandwich. He recovered from the stroke and lived another six blessed years.

Perhaps this is an extreme example of *unhelpful help*. Even so, it illustrates that trusting my deep emotions and good intentions translated into actions that were anything but helpful for my dad. In hindsight, I recognize I was motivated more by my selfish desire to make *myself* feel better about *his* situation. I wanted to *do something*. It bothered me far more than it bothered him.

This story is designed to alert you to just how tricky help can be for the helper and the "helpee."

Have you ever been on the giving (or receiving) end of unhelpful help? I call it psychopathic helpfulness (PH). I am still recovering from PH. I recognize it in others too, who, like me, have no idea they are infected. If it hadn't been for my experience with Daddy, I might have remained blind to my condition. Write this down: help is not as obvious a concept as it seems.

Have you ever tried to help someone only to have it backfire? Did you blame them for not understanding or appreciating that you meant well? Congratulations! You might be in the PH club.

Hence, helping relationships warrant ongoing clarification and forethought.

One Word, So Many Interpretations

How many ways can the word "help" be interpreted? Why are we prone to misfiring when it comes to helping others? My theory is simple and two-fold: As helpers, 1) we deeply trust our own good intentions and 2) We are darn certain we know something the "helpee" doesn't know. Because if they knew, they wouldn't be trying to change, right?

Take an informal poll of your friends. Ask how they feel about helping others. Then, ask how they feel about being helped, especially without being asked. My informal poll revealed that we tend to love to help others, especially as Christians. But when it comes to allowing others to help us do something —especially something sensitive, like losing weight—we mostly prefer to be prayed for from a distance. Generally speaking, we're prone to cross other people's boundaries—and to be on high alert when they cross ours!

What Helps You?

When the people closest to you notice you're trying to lose weight, they may want to help. But even with the best of intentions, they are more likely to guess wrong about what would help you in your weight loss journey.

Knowing your own definition of help is an important first step in reducing the number of unhelpful situations you may encounter in your weight loss journey.

By asking the simple questions below, you can identify the kind of help you desire to receive. Taking a moment to do this will help you avoid misunderstanding and conflict, which, in turn, can sabotage your progress. Can you recall a time when your weight loss efforts were affected by someone close to you? If so, then you already know how important this step is in your journey.

As you answer these questions, practice saying the answer out loud to help you clarify what works best for you.

- What is the most helpful thing anyone has ever done for me when I am trying to lose weight and live healthier?

- At home, what can I do *for myself* to make following through easier? Which of these things (or other things) could my family help me do?

- While I am at work, what can I do *for myself* to stay on track and make healthy choices? Which of these things (or other things) could my co-workers help me do?

- When I am with my friends what could I do to stay on my plan, while still having fun and enjoying the time together? How could my friends help me?

- What has caused me to stumble in the past in each of the situations above? How can I anticipate or avoid these things?

The more specifically you answer the questions, the better prepared you will be to both know what helps you, and then, be able to ask more specifically for the help you need.

You will also be prepared to gently redirect the inevitable well-meaning but unhelpful helper. Granted, if they are like me, some bricks may be required, but in most cases, the people in your life will genuinely want to help you and will receive your guidance well, especially if you deliver it well.

I used this strategy with my husband many years ago. He was tall, very fit, and had never needed to be concerned about what he ate, unlike me. As a holdover pattern from his bachelor days, he always kept a cookie jar full of store-bought oatmeal cookies.

Equally bemusing to me was his habit of taking a bite of a cookie, putting it down, and forgetting about it. At any given time, there might have been two or three partially eaten cookies randomly stationed about the house. He had no idea how hard it was for me to resist eating his abandoned cookies. I explained to him that he was inadvertently acting as a cookie pusher. I simply asked him to stop leaving the cookie carcasses lying around. Once I shared my weakness and my need for reinforcement, he was very understanding and happy to comply.

The Helpers on Your Weight Loss Journey

In addition to navigating your day-to-day relationships as you make changes and adjustments to your habits, there are two types of helping relationships that I have found to be especially beneficial in my journey: discipleship and accountability relationships.

Seek Spiritually Alive Discipleship Relationships

A woman I had met at a conference a few years ago asked to exchange contact information, and we set up a time to talk. Though I had not prayed for a discipleship relationship, the Lord knew I needed one, so He brought someone to speak into my life. Thinking back, the Lord had brought many amazing, godly women to speak into my life, and I had resisted it. This time, the Lord was showing me what discipleship looks like before I even knew what He was doing.

Diana has a deep and compelling love for and intimacy with the Lord. The Word of God drips out of her like water from a saturated sponge. It is as though His words have nearly replaced her own. When we talk and pray together, her loving spirit reveals the loving heart of God.

The time I spent with her stimulated my hunger for God's Word and my desire for increased intimacy with the Lord. I noticed a new zeal. I was running with the biggest bucket I could find to lower into the well of His Word. I sought the unrivaled security and warmth of His presence. Along the way, I was releasing less important things I had once gripped too tightly.

Before meeting Diana, I smugly felt that I was "spiritually mature." I cringe when I think about it now. I had no idea where I was spiritually. I had many blind spots that were putting me in spiritual danger. My theory is that the Lord placed me under Diana's care because He needed to rattle some idols out of my life. He knew I needed someone to come alongside me while He showed me things I needed to let go of. I hardly even knew I had idols until they began to give way around and beneath me.

Diana came alongside me in perfect Divine timing. Her prayers held me up. Her spirit-tuned ear heard my heart and wrapped it with truth from God's Word. She has fought spiritual battles for me on her knees.

While the Lord was helping me release idols and insecurities, I saw in Diana a glimpse of where I could be headed: closer to the Lord, hearing Him as never before, standing firmly on Him *in truth*—not just in my head but in my heart. I allowed what I previously stood on to crumble (albeit not so happily at the time) because I needed to learn by experience that there is no security or hope of any kind apart from the Lord Himself.

One for You?

Do you have a sister or brother in Christ who speaks into you spiritually? Consider praying that the Lord will bring someone to you or invite you into a fellowship of Godly women or men. But not just any someone or fellowship — find a discipleship relationship where you are being challenged to see what is possible a few steps ahead of you in a deeper walk of faith. Allow others to come alongside you as you take new steps into areas of deeper dependence on the Lord.

While you are praying for that Godly sister or brother to come alongside you, pray that the Lord will bring you into someone's life as well. Who can you pray for and encourage in her or his walk into deeper intimacy with God? How can you be pouring into her or him in a sacrificial way?

I believe Diana has some bruised knees and worn places on her carpet with my name on them. Lord. let me pay that forward. Let us all learn to do that for our sisters and brothers in Christ! Can you imagine the Lord's delight to answer?

Discipleship relationships are vital to the Christian community and to our spiritual health. As you are being sanctified in Christ, seek the company of believers who call you forward into deeper intimacy with Him and deeper into His Word. You will know you are in the right place if it makes you feel the way Peter might have felt when he said to Jesus, "Lord bid me come to you on the water."

And Jesus said, "Come!"

Seek Effective Accountability Relationships

Just as the word "help" can mean different things to different people, so can the word "accountability." *Good* accountability relationships are a necessary part of any long-term change journey. Numerous studies confirm improved results when social support is present. I love it when science "proves" what God designed to be true. We need each other.

Accountability relationships could also be discipleship relationships, but I prefer to keep them separate. An accountability relationship is more mutual and more practical in nature.

Of the accountability relationships I have had, some have not worked well. Finding a good fit required trial and error. My best accountability partnership is still ongoing and has been working fabulously for several years. It is fun, supportive, and helps keep me on track.

The following "DOs" and "DON'Ts" of accountability will help you get the most power out of your partnership.

My Axioms of Accountability: DOs and DON'Ts
Do:

- **Pray first.** Pray for the partner the Lord has for you. How can you be a blessing to your partner? Ask the Lord to teach you how to serve and support your partner from the heart and with His wisdom.

- **Partner with a spiritually committed person of the same gender.** It is vitally important that your accountability partner shares your faith. All your efforts to lose weight will be taking place in the context of your relationship with the Lord, your desire to please Him, and your effort to bring your life into submission to Him. An unbeliever may respect your faith but might not understand the role that sanctification, God's ongoing work in your heart, plays in the outcome you are seeking. There is a big difference between self-improvement and self-surrender.

- **Pre-define what successful accountability looks like.** Whether you realize it or not, you have a preconceived notion of what the success of the relationship means to you. Spell it out and tweak it into something well-defined (but flexible), mutually beneficial, and fun. Convey this to your partner so that she or he knows what you need and can respond.

- **Define, specifically, what you want to be held accountable for**. Mainly, know what you need. I know where I'm weak, where I need to focus more effort to fight past weakness, and to keep my weaknesses before God in prayer. I trust my accountability partner to support me in my areas of vulnerability.

    Examples may include:

    o   Not eating after a specific time.
    o   Reporting your weight.
    o   Waking up early for time with the Lord.
    o   Taking 30 minutes for afternoon prayer.
    o   Taking a certain number of steps each day.
    o   Logging food in a food-tracking app.
    o   Journaling daily.
    o   Memorizing Scripture.

- **Plan how to communicate with your partner** I like to report my progress to my partner by text, as does she. Do you prefer to communicate by phone or meet in person? Make sure your preferences match your partner's preferences. I have been in accountability relationships where my partner preferred the phone. Talking on the phone is my least preferred form of accountability communication. Because of that, the partnership was a mismatch and ultimately fizzled.

- **Set up a mutually agreed upon schedule.** My current accountability partner likes to provide a detailed report twice a week. There are some areas I like to report on almost every day. We both initiate our own reporting in. If one of us delays, we reach out. We celebrate each other's wins and exhort each other to pick up, dust off, and soldier on when we stumble.

Don't:

- **Don't ask for accountability for something you are not willing to do.** Don't place your accountability partner in the awful position of being your mom, babysitter, or police. If you do, you aren't seeking accountability. Instead, you are seeking a warden that you don't really want and are unwilling to cooperate with. Start with actions you are willing to commit to and hold yourself accountable for. Then, build from there. Saying what you will do and doing it will make you a good partner. Find one who does the same.

- **Don't assume you already know your partner's needs.** Be careful to allow your partner to define what they want to be held accountable for. Don't presume what you *think* she/he needs. I may think I know what my partner "ought to do," but she has proven over and over that she knows what is best for her. I listen to what she asks for and offer accountability in the way she has asked. She does the same for me.

- **Don't choose more than two things (three at the most) you want to be held accountable for.** We don't have the capacity to change more than a few actions, behaviors, or thoughts at a time. Further, having too many issues to keep up with will undermine the accountability relationship by making it too cumbersome for you and your partner to manage.

- **Don't "set it and forget it."** Accountability relationships need to be fed, nurtured, and allowed to breathe and grow. They must be dynamic. My partner and I periodically ask, "Is this still working for you?" If it has become stale, we tweak it, and it comes to life again. Perhaps this is why it has lasted for many years.

- **Don't stay in an accountability relationship that doesn't fit or work. Be sure to end it with kindness and grace.** Encourage your potential partner to join you in considering a trial period. If either senses that it would not be a good fit, then clarify what you need. If you can't reach a compromise, then you can both agree to continue looking for a better match.

I hope these "axioms" will help you find the partner or partners you need to make the journey of long-term change and permanent weight loss together.

Reflections

Community plays a much bigger role in your success than you may realize. The people in our lives are intertwined in ways we may not have noticed until we start making changes to our routines.

It's also difficult to anticipate how much each person in your life counts on you doing what you have always done in the way you have always done it. It gives them comfort. When you make changes in your life, they'll not only notice but may even be affected in ways you don't foresee. Be patient and gracious and prepare in advance to help smooth potential rough spots that your weight loss journey may create for them. They may, in turn, be more eager to do what you need to support you.

Here are some questions to help you

Questions

This is a longer Questions section, so you may want to move through each series of questions in individual sessions. Don't push yourself to rush through these questions, but take the time to think through and absorb each one.

Who is My Community?

1. As you think about the people in your life and the type of influence they have, make a note of them below. Who is:

- The nutritional gatekeeper (the one who does most of the shopping/cooking)?

- The food preference monster (the one who is so picky that it always affects the menu)?

- The saboteur (the one who brings you treats even knowing you are trying to lose weight)?

- The food police (the one who knows you're trying and questions your food choices)?

- Any other types?

2. Do any of these titles apply to you? Which ones?

3. Whose lives are intertwined enough with yours, that you influence every day?

4. On a Scale of 1-10, with *1* being easy and *10* being very difficult, how hard is it for you to ask for help?

5. List some of the reasons why it is hard for you to ask for help.

Looking at Family, Inner Circle, and Church

1. List the people in your **family** (and/or who you live with) and the ways each person **supports** or **challenges** your weight loss efforts.

2. List the people in your **inner circle** and the ways each person **supports** or **challenges** your weight loss efforts.

3. List the people you are closest to in your **church** and the ways each person **supports** or **challenges** your weight loss efforts.

4. As you think about these separate groups, who do you desire the most help from?

5. Write out who you see as your most important allies in this journey and where/how you anticipate them helping you.

Identifying the Kind of Help You Need

Read Ecclesiastes 4:9-12.

Two are better than one, because they have a good reward for their toil. ¹⁰ For if they fall, one will lift up his fellow. But woe to him who is alone when he falls and has not another to lift him up! ¹¹ Again, if two lie together, they keep warm, but how can one keep warm alone? ¹² And though a man might prevail against one who is alone, two will withstand him—a threefold cord is not quickly broken.

1. List the reasons from the passage that Solomon, the writer, declares it is better not to be alone.

2. How does the same reasoning apply to you in your efforts to break free from the bondage of weight issues?

3. Do you have people in your life who have helped you get back on track when you have strayed —in any way, whether health or otherwise?

   a.) If you do, mention them here:

   b.) What kinds of things have they done, and how specifically did they help?

4. If you don't have people like this in your life, reflect on why. (For me, at times I have avoided accountability and vulnerability. Other times, I hadn't done my part to develop those relationships.)

Giving the Help Others Need
Read Galatians 6:1-2, 9-10.

Brothers, if anyone is caught in any transgression, you who are spiritual should restore him in a spirit of gentleness. Keep watch on yourself, lest you too be tempted. ² Bear one another's burdens, and so fulfill the law of Christ.

And let us not grow weary of doing good, for in due season we will reap, if we do not give up. ¹⁰ So then, as we have opportunity, let us do good to everyone, and especially to those who are of the household of faith.

1. In what ways is it difficult is it to live out these verses? Explain your answer

2. How would you react to another sibling in Christ coming to you in the spirit of holding you accountable or restoring you?

3. Why would Paul think this is so important that he instructs the church in Galatia to do it for each other? What does it accomplish?

4. List ideas of what you can be doing today to fulfill what Paul is asking of the Galatians. Perhaps you are already doing some of these things. If so, write those as well.

5. Name several people that you see regularly —that live in your household or that you work with and worship with. What can you do to offer them encouragement in their walk with Christ? Give examples of how you can encourage each person.

5. Write a prayer asking the Lord to help you develop a spirit of endurance in serving the community of believers surrounding you.

Final Word

I hope by now, you can appreciate why losing weight permanently is much more than a physical or even psychological change. It requires the transforming work of Christ in our hearts. It is a spiritual change process that will unfold into changes in your choices, your relationship with food, and your health. These will be byproducts of the healing work the Lord wants to do in your life.

By looking at change from a spiritual rather than a behavioral perspective, we rightly place ourselves in His hands to transform us.

Ask the Lord to help you see your heart clearly and to give you the wisdom and willingness to move forward. Then, do your part to move forward with Him. When the Lord transforms our hearts, change becomes possible in a way we could never accomplish with mere willpower. Genuine change occurs only with God's power and our cooperation, and it needs to be reinforced within a community of believers.

There is more to come in the *I Once Was Fat* series. For more information about "Stop Dieting for Life" or our online course, check us out at StopDietingforLife.com

Notes

1. Prochaska, James O., and John C. Norcross. *Changing for Good: The Revolutionary Program That Explains the Six Stages of Change and Teaches You How to Free Yourself from Bad Habits.* New York: W. Morrow, 1994.

2. Piper, John. *When I Don't Desire God: How to Fight For Joy.* Leicester, England: Crossway Books, 2004.

3. Chan, Francis, and Danae Yankoski. *Crazy Love: Overwhelmed by a Relentless God.* Colorado Springs, Colo.: David C. Cook, 2008.

4. Zacharias, Ravi K. *Jesus Among Other Gods: The Absolute Claims of the Christian Message.* Nashville, TN: Thomas Nelson, 2000.

About the Author

Laura Fulford is the founder and creator of **Stop Dieting for Life™**, a Christian weight loss program. A graduate of Wake Forest University (B.S. in Exercise Science), she works with groups and individuals, helping them abandon old food and weight strongholds and re-align with God's design for eating and living. The **Stop Dieting for Life™** course is available online at stopdietingforlife.com.

Made in the USA
Columbia, SC
24 May 2020